The Red Button

Creating Good Choices at the End of Life for People Living with Dementia

Richard Fenker, PhD

978-0-9894600-2-6 (paperback)
978-0-9894600-3-3 (ebook)

Published by Cimarron International Publishing
865A Camino Los Abuelos
Galisteo, NM 87540
(505) 820-1686
Rich@RichardFenker.com

Praise for

The Red Button

This powerful book speaks to an issue I have struggled with ever since my Alzheimer's diagnosis. I am living with a kind of pain and suffering that no one seems to understand. Everyone deserves a good life, from birth until death. Planning a pain-free death should be as important as planning an enjoyable vacation. Those of us who are living with a dementia-related illness should have the right to choose how their life should come to a peaceful end.

Living with Alzheimer's, my fear is that at the end of life I will be helpless, suffering, and unable to die with dignity. The Red Button *gave me the power and knowledge to make good choices now and later.*

Brian LeBlanc (living with Alzheimer's since 2014)
Dementia Advocate / Keynote Speaker /
National and International Alzheimer's Advisory Board Member

It's a Wonderful Life *is one of my favorite movies. How sad to live that life and yet, because of the stigma and misunderstanding associated with dementia, endure the opposite when dying. This wonderful book is brave enough and compassionate enough to offer options for people with dementia to experience a more dignified death.*

Michael Belleville (living with dementia since 2013)
Board Member, MA/NH Alzheimer's Association / Technology
Committee Member and Podcast Manager, Dementia Action Alliance

The Red Button *is of utmost importance for anyone living with a dementia diagnosis or caring for someone with one.*

End-of-life decisions are very controversial but must be faced, especially by anyone with a diagnosis of dementia. I have seen suicide at young ages by people living with dementia leaving young children behind, and I have seen my father, an Alzheimer's victim, lose every shred of dignity as he failed progressively beyond hope long beyond what I hope I face as I am living with vascular dementia. Let us all die with dignity.

Paulan Gordon
(living with Vascular Dementia) Author: *Vascular Dementia: An Inside Perspective* / Board Member, Dementia Action Alliance

Dr. Richard Fenker, Emeritus Professor of Psychology, author, photographer, and technologist is a longtime member and friend of the Dementia Action Alliance. He shares our vision of a society in which individuals living with dementia are ENGAGED, ENABLED, and EMPOWERED and fully included in all matters that affect them. In his latest book, The Red Button, *Dr. Fenker shares a caring and compelling case for those living with dementia to determine what a good death would be and discuss and document those wishes with family, medical and legal representatives while they still can. Over 50 million people in the world have dementia. With only 10% receiving hospice, most live for years with poor life quality and then die without dignity. This is a problem we have chosen to avoid.*

A must-read for all concerned!!

Jackie Pinkowitz, M.Ed.
Board Chair, Dementia Action Alliance

While the concept of a "good death" is widely accepted in society, within the community of people living with dementia, it is largely absent. Here, choices that can lead to a timely and dignified death are rare. In his new book, Richard Fenker addresses the challenging issue of creating good choices at the end of life for people with dementia and other disorders that impact thinking. His philosophy matches that of our organization: "Every person living with dementia has the right to live a good life for as long as possible, to live free from the dementia stigma that is common in our society, and to experience a 'good death' by dying in a timely and dignified manner."

Karen Love
CEO, Dementia Action Alliance

This important book addresses a problem I deal with every day in my work as a counselor for people living with dementia and their families: how to overcome the fear of ending life in a helpless, painful, and undignified manner. Dr. Fenker's "Red Button" program and its recommendations are certain to bring relief to a lot of families and caregivers. Talking about our wishes at the end of our lives is uncomfortable for most of us, even those of us whose professions are focused on the elderly. Trying to ascertain the realistic wishes once a loved one is living with dementia is often very tricky. The tendency is to push it off into the future.

Thank you, Dr. Fenker, for making the process more transparent and much easier for everyone to understand and implement.

Jytte Lokvig, PhD
Alzheimer's & Dementia Counselor and Educator /
Author, *Alzheimer's A to Z, Successful Caregiving*
(and five other related books)

For Dick and the many others
who long for the option of
a timely and dignified death

Contents

Introduction

Why You Need to Read This Book If You or a Loved One Have Dementia

1. One hundred million people globally are living with Alzheimer's disease and other dementias, Parkinson's, Huntington's, and other conditions that involve a degenerative brain disorder that limits options at the end of life.
2. Many of these people, perhaps including yourself, will not enjoy the blessing of a "good death" or other options, such as hospice care, that are available to most people at the end of their life.
3. Medical interventions at the end of life can prolong life but often come with a high cost and diminished quality of life. Family, caregivers, and medical professionals will make these decisions (perhaps guided by medical directives), not the individuals with dementia.
4. The concept of *pain and suffering*, while well understood with many diseases and medical conditions, is

not well understood with dementia. A passive, vegetative state with virtually no functioning memory is likely to be considered benign, not an extreme form of suffering.

5. *The Red Button* is about offering choices to people living with dementia and other diseases to minimize pain and suffering and to avoid extending life beyond the bounds of acceptable life quality.
6. A "good death" is a normal part of every good life, and living with dementia does not mean giving up either of these. Living well today supports dying well because most "good deaths" are simply natural extensions of a life lived with quality and choice.
7. Can a person with dementia, judged to be mentally noncompetent, make a choice about hospice or euthanasia at the end of life? Or will this choice need to be made by family or others? Can we even tell when a person with Alzheimer's, for example, is experiencing pain and suffering?
8. *The Red Button* seeks to expand our current definitions of pain and suffering to include those mental and physical conditions associated with dementia and other neurological disorders, especially near the end of life.
9. *The Red Button* addresses all of these issues and many others. Its goal is to make choices about the end of life available to those who currently lack choice so that their deaths are timely, dignified, and involve a minimum of pain and suffering.

The Line

Finding the line between life and death is like catching a ghost, bare-handed. Perhaps it is present and real, perhaps not. When it is sudden and sharp and etched into our lives like the crack of a whip, we understand. We get it, gasp, and grieve in acknowledgment. When it is blurred by time and ends in a gradual and expected decline with loved ones present, we celebrate with a familiar eulogy and the peace that a good death brings. But frequently this is all an illusion. Death is a process, typically years in its development, and is cloaked in the denials that are convenient for the living.

Pain and suffering are often part of death and the descent from "living a full life" into the chasm of uncertainty that the line represents. Because fear and denial are also part of this journey, the role of suffering may very well be to help bring reality back into focus. Because we do understand suffering, experiencing suffering in ourselves or others can help us find the line, lost in our denials, and denote it more clearly. This is part of the reason that ending a life filled with pain is acceptable and appropriate in many cultures.

As you might expect, however, the ghost is more complicated than a clearly delineated boundary with life on one side and death on the other. Living with late-stage dementia, the line is now an endless series of dawns and nights filled with blurred memories that never quite come into focus. Life, on one side of the line, is present in chunks or moments of reality, experienced like gulps of air inhaled as you struggle to breathe. Living and memory are present for a moment and then gone, a cruel illusion. We know that music and other stimuli can wake you from this sleep, but only for a brief period. And pain, what about pain? No one knows because your Alzheimer's mind is uncharted territory.

Where is the line between life and death? Have you actually died already and confused your caregivers and physicians by marginally manifesting the physical signs of life? Now the line is not a simple barrier to be crossed in a single leap, dying quietly in your sleep one night. No, it is a chasm of unknown depth where you may wander, helpless, for years, lost and suffering. From above, occasional shouts of "attaboy" penetrate the darkness and perhaps the familiar music in a therapy program makes you smile. But where, oh where, is the line? And when will you cross it? Are you ready, if this option existed? We would like to help but the fog is too thick. We cannot see you. We cannot hear you. I am so sorry.

Part I

What Is the Red Button?

1

Everyone Needs a Red Button

This is a book about understanding and exercising the choices we have for ending our lives in a timely and dignified manner. The Red Button sits at the boundary between a life lived with quality and limited inconvenience and one lived with unbearable pain and suffering. Pushing the Red Button is a cry for help.

This is a book about creating choices for people with dementia at the end of life so that their deaths are timely, dignified, and involve a minimum of pain and suffering. As you will see, for many reasons this is a complex topic burdened by our fear of death as well as the stigma and general lack of understanding of dementia. For these individuals, the Red Button sits at the boundary between a life lived with quality, limited inconvenience, and pain or discomfort followed by a timely death, and one extended unnecessarily or lived in a fog with the possibility of unbearable pain and suffering over a long period.

Think of the Red Button as an emergency switch, waiting somewhere in the journey of your life, that can communicate a single message: *It's time to get off of this train.* Pushing the Red Button is a cry for help. It's a silent statement of the fact that the pain and suffering you or someone else is experiencing is too much to bear and that you choose death—or at least not to prolong life—in your current condition.

Everyone needs the options that having a Red Button creates at the end of life, even though most people will never need to use one. Herein lies the core conundrum: the more likely you are to need the choices offered by having a Red Button, the less likely you are to have one! Most of us will die normal, benign "good deaths" surrounded by family and friends and a minimum of pain and suffering. People living with dementia or other conditions judged to impact mental competence, however, will long for a Red Button but not have access to one because of their condition.

Normal mind = CHOICES.
Handicapped mind = NO CHOICES.

Dementia-related deaths tend to be long, extended affairs that can last for years and be very stressful for the individuals and their caregivers. Mostly they represent deaths that offer quite limited options and a strong likelihood that you, the person with dementia, will be caught in the medical community's focus on extending life regardless of its quality or your family's conflicts over end-of-life decisions absent traditional concrete guidelines.

What is most important here is that you have lost your choice. You will not have the option to select hospice or an assisted death, if the latter is even legal in your state or country. You will not be able to communicate your inevitable pain and suffering because of your mental disability—even though it may be obvious to caregivers and staff. The choices you really want, those that are available to most others—to live a quality life now and, when it is time, to avoid unnecessary pain and suffering and embrace death in your own terms—are missing.

One of the biggest challenges here is to define *pain and suffering* in this context. Is living passively in a vegetative state pain and suffering? What about memory loss so severe that you no longer remember family and friends? What about constant fear and frustration? We don't know, and because we don't know, there is little agreement. The 1–10 pain scale doesn't help much here, although the concept of pain is still extremely relevant.

Another big challenge is communication. More people have returned from the moon to communicate their experience than have returned from the black hole of late-stage dementia to describe what this is like, from the inside out. A survey of my friends currently living with Alzheimer's, in the early stages or midstages, found eleven of twelve wanting to start hospice when 24-hour care was required and they could no longer recognize family.

Can a person with late-stage dementia communicate meaningfully about a concept such as death or hospice? If so, how would this process work? What would it take for you or a physician or an attorney to accept the communication as real? These are important questions that we will explore in later chapters.

Finally, while we understand physical death, when the body's organs stop functioning, and have a vast array of tools and medicines available to arrest or delay such deaths, we know little about the death of the mind and normal human consciousness. Could the mind fail in the same way other major organs fail, making a quality life unattainable while we in our ignorance force physical life to continue, because this is what medicine does?

Ultimately, living a quality life and enjoying a good death is about choice. Regardless of your current circumstances, my goal in writing this book is to give you or others in your family the choice to understand, create, and push your own Red Button if this is ever needed. Ironically, as you will see, these choices are much more about your life than your death.

2

Dementia and the Red Button

Many people living with dementia, Parkinson's, Huntington's, and other diseases that involve a degenerative brain disorder have limited options at the end of life. Most, perhaps including yourself, will not enjoy the blessing of a good death. They have lost their choices.

One hundred million people globally are living with dementia, Parkinson's, Huntington's, and other diseases that involve a degenerative brain disorder that limits choices at the end of life. Many of these people, perhaps including yourself, will not enjoy the blessing of a good death or other options, such as hospice care, that are available to most people at the end of their life. Medical interventions at the end of life can prolong life but often come with a high cost, including a diminished quality of life. Family, caregivers, and medical professionals will make these decisions (perhaps guided by medical directives), not the individuals with dementia.

The concept of pain and suffering, while accepted and measured (with the pain scale) for many diseases and medical conditions, is not well understood with dementia and other disorders that impact mental functioning. A passive, vegetative state with virtually no functioning memory is likely to be considered an unfortunate but comfortable condition, not an extreme form of suffering.

The Red Button is about offering choices to people living with dementia to minimize pain and suffering and to avoid extending life beyond the bounds of acceptable life quality. Can a person with dementia, judged to be mentally incompetent, make a choice about hospice or euthanasia at the end of life? Will this choice need to be made by family or others? Can we even tell when a person with Alzheimer's, for example, is experiencing pain and suffering?

The Red Button addresses all of these issues and many others that make choices about the end of life available to those who currently lack choice. *The Red Button* seeks to expand our current definitions of pain and suffering to include those mental and physical conditions associated with dementia and other disorders, especially near the end of life. Do Not Resuscitate is a clear and widely understood Red Button available now to everyone. Could such a clear boundary exist for someone with dementia?

3

An Example of a Red Button

A Message to My Family and Friends:

I am asking, once more, for your help. We have finished my medical directives and outlined the content of the conversation that we will record on video so that there is no doubt about my intent. Perhaps the most challenging part of that video will be our discussion of the Red Button and the specific conditions that might lead you to hasten ending my life because of the pain and suffering I am experiencing. I have some guidelines for you to use in making this decision but that is as far as I can go. This is new territory for both of us.

At the point in time when the Red Button has relevance, it is not very likely to have any cognitive or logical significance to me. The emotional part of my brain may be able to communicate with you, so you can hear my cry for help, but this is largely an unknown. It is possible that my pain and suffering will be so obvious that it helps support your decision, but perhaps not. Despite the uncertainty here, I am asking for you to do your best to understand and, if we reach the point where my suffering is past the thresholds we have discussed, do all you can to hasten the end of my life—for which I will be eternally grateful.

I will say it in our video conversation, but I want to repeat it now. I believe in the fullness of life and in the importance of overcoming difficulties, including pain and suffering, until they are resolved. In the case of my dementia, however, there will come a point when my battle has ended, when no amount of willpower on my part or love and assistance from you will make a difference. There will be no meaning to my life or point in my continued living other than as a blip on a medical chart. When these circumstances arise, please hear me: ***I no longer wish to continue to live****. I view my death as the most natural, appropriate, and timely conclusion to a life already well-lived. I am blessed by your support in helping implement my wishes here and want you to understand that in doing so you are loving me in the most important and powerful of ways, while I am powerless. Please also know that there is no guilt or shame in your decision to speed the end of my life. You are offering me the comfort and support that can* *only come at this time through peace and closure. For these things I am very grateful.*

This simple request for help, as a part of your conversation about death and the limits of living with the pain and suffering of dementia, is a profoundly powerful statement made at a time while you still are healthy and capable of guiding the important decisions about your life. Know that it is a risky statement because the decisions you are asking others to make in the future are filled with unknowns. You will be asking family and other caregivers to take a giant leap of faith to interpret your condition, which may not be obvious. In asking for the Red Button you are saying that you are fully committed to accepting this uncertainty and willing to live and die according to the consequences that will follow.

Your mantra is clear and unwavering. When your pain and suffering is intense and when there is no path forward toward recovery or significant improvement, you are choosing to hasten the end of your life by whatever means are ethically, legally, and practically appropriate. You are also asking your family and friends and caregivers to support you by recognizing your distress and honoring the commitments made to you at the time your conversation about death was recorded. It will take strength and determination on their part to respect your wishes, because, in doing so, they will need to overcome the social norms that currently guide deaths for people living with dementia and the reservations they may have because of their own beliefs and understanding of death.

Life, with the opportunity to live fully, is an enormous blessing; death, with the option of dying in a timely and peaceful manner, is the same. You are asking your care providers to temporarily suspend their fear of death and society's reservations about having frank and healthy conversations about death, to join you at a time when you cannot make choices, and to give you the gift of ending your pain and suffering as soon as it is appropriate.

Part II

Why Do You Need a Red Button?

4

Endings . . . A Few Examples

The ideal ending to life that most people imagine is to die peacefully at home, with a minimum of pain and discomfort, surrounded by family and friends. Reality does not often match this ideal, especially for people with dementia.

Common endings to life are usually benign but not always. Here are a few examples culled from obituaries and personal knowledge:

- George Bush lived a long and healthy life. At age 93, after a bout with pneumonia, and the failure of several major systems that prevented eating, the decision was made to not provide life support. He died, while sleeping, 48 hours later, with his family at his bedside.

- Dick, age 78, had early stage to midstage Alzheimer's disease. He lived life fully, was still driving, and if you spent an evening with him, his dementia might not be noticed. He feared the ending he could see coming, however, and took his own life.

- Betty was a teenager in Texas when she started using drugs. Marijuana, coke, and other recreational drugs soon led to crack, heroin, and opioids. After ten years on the street, with multiple attempts at rehabilitation and good family support, she died of an overdose.

- Emilou died in her sleep of heart failure at age 103 in a memory-care facility. For the last five years of her life, although she was not experiencing physical pain, she needed 24-hour care and no longer recognized family and friends.

- Martha lived a full, healthy life with family and friends. It included the inconveniences of aging and occasional short periods of depression, but nothing more. After the loss of a spouse, she elected euthanasia after a broken hip required surgery.

- These obituaries and the dozens more you can find in any Sunday paper are designed to tell the stories of death with a soft brush that blurs the pain and hardship. While we understand this and accept it, this softening clashes with the harsh realities the Alzheimer's Association presents for dementia-related deaths:

> A diagnosis of Alzheimer's disease will bring an extended period of pain and suffering to you and your family for many years. In the later stages you will most likely not recognize your family and friends, you will need 24-hour care, and feelings of anxiety or mental confusion and anger may persist.

This vision of death with Alzheimer's or other dementias runs so counter to the soft versions of death we read in obituaries that it provokes the fear and stigma that we see in society today. It is scary for many reasons, but one of the biggest is that, with Alzheimer's, you will be without choices. Your expectations about the end of life will have plummeted from options for a good death to what physicians and others describe as "living in hell for many years."

The ideal ending that most people imagine is to die peacefully at home, with a minimum of pain and discomfort, surrounded by family and friends. What happens when this is not available? What about the end of your life? What options would you choose, if you had the choice to decide?

5

The Myth of the Good Death

Most people expect to die a good death with an ending like the ones described in chapter 4, at home surrounded by family. Yet more than 50 percent of deaths take place in hospitals or other treatment facilities—and this is especially true for those living with dementia.

Both culturally and practically many people embrace the idea of living well, living big, living fully or living the good life. The idea of a good death is also a widely accepted cultural myth. The National Institute on Aging's definition is this:

> A good death is one that comes quickly and painlessly with full awareness of family, friends and shared life experiences, and the opportunity to say goodbye. A good death is one that is preceded by a

good life up until the time of death, a life that is lived fully, healthfully and joyfully with a minimum of suffering and inconvenience due to aging or disease or financial considerations.

Part of the mystique of the good death is that it will take place at home and, at the moment of death, the person will be surrounded by family and friends. The reality here is that over 50 percent of deaths in the United States take place in hospitals, many after expensive, invasive medical procedures are used to extend life. Also, while dying at home may be the ideal, such deaths are not necessarily timely, painless, or without many of the other conditions associated with a good death.

The core issue here is not really whether your death will be in a hospital or at home; it is about choice. You get to have a voice in when you are ready for death and, ideally, about some of the associated conditions. As you will see, many people, including most of those living with dementia, are currently denied this choice.

The purpose of the Red Button is not to somehow fix the complex problems associated with deaths that don't fit the mold or definition of good deaths. Rather it is intended to address the problem of the quality of life for anyone nearing death who currently, for whatever reason, lacks choice—especially the choice to terminate life or at least not prolong pain and suffering. If the idea of ending life sounds too strong for you or conflicts with your beliefs, remember that the guidelines for doing this under certain conditions already exist as part of your medical directives and are accepted by over 80 percent of the population.

How do you feel about a good death? Is it important for you to have this option, despite living with dementia?

6

Why Does a Good Death Matter?

A good death matters because it is more a statement about how you are living life at the end than about death.

In the simplest terms, a good death matters to you because it represents not just your death, the ending, but also how you lived your life. A good death is about the *quality of life* at *the end of life* and, yes, in some cases the end of life can last for years! The stigma of Alzheimer's and other dementias often prevents us from recognizing that people with dementia can live ten or more years after diagnosis and spend much of this time living fully and happily.

A good death helps to bring the story of your life to a close with dignity and a special kind of integrity that refuses to undermine how you lived. When we remember most of our family and friends who are deceased, we remember their lives. The moment of their death and associated details are but a footnote that grows quickly more irrelevant with the passage of time.

Living for years, until death, with extensive pain or other kinds of suffering or with any other condition (including living in a vegetative state) that diminishes life quality—this is not living a good life or a good death. Unless this is your choice, it is not okay.

Would you be willing to extend your pain and suffering to add precious time with your family and have important conversations with loved ones? Perhaps, but that is a choice you can make. When you are ready for death, you should also have the option of choosing a Red Button.

Ask anyone living with dementia today if they want the option to have a Red Button to end pain and suffering at the end of life—they will say yes. This is an important part of living a full life with quality. This is an important part of their story.

7

How Did People with Dementia Lose the Option for a Good Death?

They never had this option. Diseases that impact mental functioning, such as dementia, carry the burden of a huge stigma in our society. Expectations shaped by this stigma, medical professionals, and the Alzheimer's Association are that the process of dying will be long, painful, and devastating for the individual and their family.

People with dementia did not lose this option, they never had it.

The medical establishment feels helpless in the face of a disease that has no cure, and they pass this negativity and sense of hopelessness on to individuals with an Alzheimer's diagnosis. Mental illness and diseases that relate to mental functioning such as dementia carry the burden of a huge stigma in our society that compromises those living with and dying with the disease.

Our boundaries for what is okay or normal mentally define a very narrow slice of reality. You are normal only when you share the same limited, logical, verbal view of the world—and can communicate this view to others with words. The heart of this world view is simply shared agreements about reality.

People who cannot speak and verbally confirm these shared agreements about the world—what is green or red, what is correct or incorrect, what meaning specific words convey, what they want or don't want—are put into a special category: mentally handicapped. The stigma and the practical reality of living with dementia (which quickly impacts linear, logical, verbal processes) means you will be quickly placed into this category as the disease progresses.

Since a good death is much more about living a quality life until the end than about dying, the judgment that you are mentally handicapped means you will also lose choices here. Society is not going to quickly stretch to become inclusive in its understanding of dementia and the rights of people living with dementia. The dementia community will need to do the stretching and the educating and the pushing to affirm these rights.

The Red Button is an affirmation of the importance of choices around pain and suffering at the end of life for those with dementia and other disorders that affect the mind, regardless of diminishing verbal skills, memory loss, and other cognitive limitations. Everyone with dementia wants the option of a good death. Let's give it back to them.

8

Who Owns Your Death?

The battle for control over your death will involve your family, your estate, the medical profession, the law, and your place of residence, as a start! Living with dementia you will have very little say unless you act now, while your voice can be heard.

We know end-of-life choices are limited for people with dementia, but the story does not end there. Many people face some limits in their choices because it may not be clear, when it matters most, who is in control. As you will see, medical directives can be powerful, helpful guides here, but not always. Ultimately the decision will be in the hands of a family member or advocate who may lack the courage and will to make the tough decisions you want.

The shift from a focus on living to a focus on avoiding death through surgery, medications, radiation treatment, or other procedures can be very stressful and create a reduced quality of life.

In our society it is clear that, to a large degree, we own our lives and our physicians own our deaths. In one session, my dad's new physician at his residential care facility canceled half of the prescriptions my dad had taken for years. That was the beginning of the end for his health and eventually led to his death.

The toughest decisions here often come not in the context of death, but of continued living in the diminished circumstances that Alzheimer's or Parkinson's or even cancer can create. Can you continue to live at home or is a residential care facility or hospital needed? Your pain and frustration are evident. What steps are needed to address these issues? Person-centered care facilities offer a precious lifeline here for folks living with dementia because they get to the root causes of the pain and frustration, but they represent only a small fraction of the available facilities. Decisions about any of these topics will be challenging for your family and other caregivers.

As the conversation shifts from concerns about living to those associated with your death, it is apparent that there are many stakeholders:

1. You
2. Your family and caregivers
3. The medical establishment
4. Your estate and the attorneys managing it
5. Your church and other organizations you support

6. Your social status
7. Chance

Things are complicated. Given the complexity of ownership here, even in the best of circumstances, decisions near the end of life often have a good deal of uncertainty associated with them. You can cut through much of this complexity by making good choices now in several key areas, discussed further in Part III.

9

Pushing and Letting Go

In the first stage of life we are constantly pushing, physically and mentally, to grow, survive, compete, earn a living, raise a family, achieve our goals, and much more. In the second half of life we will need to begin letting go of the many things accumulated in the first half.

To fully appreciate choices made near the end of life, we need to understand the two main cycles that guide each half of our lives. When I use the word *choice*, it suggests a measure of control and the ability to "make things happen" late in life or in connection with your death. While this is partially true, decisions made later in life and the kinds of control you can manifest are much more about gently guiding or allowing events to occur, not forcing or making them occur.

The Two Cycles

PUSHING: In the first stage of life we are constantly pushing. Pushing physically and mentally to grow, survive, compete, earn a living, raise a family, achieve our goals, and much more; pushing to control the world by bending it in the directions of our choosing; pushing to make things happen.

The fear of death and of diseases such as Alzheimer's that diminishes our control of the world is strong and pervasive during this period in our life.

LETTING GO: The second half of life, ending (of course) in death, is much more about letting go. Regardless of how successful you have been in terms of jobs, family, money, fame, and all of the things people strive for, sooner or later you will begin to turn loose many of these things and allow the sharp boundaries and judgments that once defined you to blur. This may occur in the middle of your life, or, without the ability to relinquish the need to fight every day to survive, you can continue pushing almost to the very end.

In most lives there is a symmetry as we pass from being a helpless infant through all of the stages of ego—learning, striving, working, competing—and eventually return at death to that same open, helpless, nonjudgmental place where we began. Physicians, caregivers, and hospice staff who deal regularly with death where pain and suffering doesn't exist or is minimized all describe the serenity and the beauty of this transition into a natural, end-of-life place of spirit and joy as well as sadness.

A dementia diagnosis doesn't change the rules, but it does impact the timing. Living with dementia accelerates the transition from ego to letting go and forces it to happen rather than allowing it to occur as a natural, voluntary process that comes with aging, learning, and other life conditions such as retirement.

The shock of a dementia diagnosis sends a ripple through all of the parts of your mind used to controlling reality because suddenly you know this will not continue. Your ego will survive but the very heart of this ego—conscious, goal-driven behavior—is now compromised. You will be dependent on others and not necessarily in a good way. You must let go, yet your dilemma is that dementia won't let this happen fully either. You are caught in the often frustrating process of trying to survive in a world that is still filled with demands—to eat, to bathe, to communicate, to get by—while rendering you helpless at the same time. The best of the person-centered treatment programs offer many kinds of support for letting go, but the demands of everyday living plus the stigma of dementia and the conflicts this creates can keep you pushing.

In this context, the Red Button represents a call for help to end life when its quality has diminished to the point where you can no longer survive with dignity, joy, awareness of the world around you and other qualities you judge to be important. The Red Button is a precaution, put in place during a healthy stage of your life, that in the late stages of dementia may be merely a landmark to those watching, but for you it screams of the need for resolution and closure.

10

Hospice and Palliative Care

Hospice offers a gentle and widely used path to the end of life when you judge it to be time to end the pain and suffering.

What is hospice care? The Catholic Hospice Center defines hospice:

> Hospice care is designed to provide support to you and your loved ones during the final phase of life. Hospice care focuses on your comfort and provides a better quality of life, with the goal to enable you to have an alert, pain-free life and live each day as fully as possible.

Comfort, reducing pain, enhancing the quality of life—all of these concepts are important for anyone, with or without dementia, in the last stages of life. Notice that questions about the person's awareness and ability to make the choice to start hospice are buried in the definition; but, in most cases, it is assumed that the individual or the individual with the family's help can make this decision from a personal and legal perspective, with the guidance of a physician. Dementia adds a gray area here, as the conditions necessary to offer hospice often don't apply.

Timing is key. To start hospice, the team (the person, physician, family, and others) must agree that the individual will likely die within the next six months. Why? Because the focus now is comfort, not prolonging life, and many medical procedures that can be used to prolong life will no longer apply. However, if the individual is not near death based on their physical condition, then there is no legal or medical basis for starting hospice.

Dad started hospice after a bout with congestive heart failure but was "evicted" after six months when his condition improved. As you will see in the next chapter, people living with dementia do have limited access to hospice care at the very end of life as major organs and body systems begin to fail; but they can also live years in limbo, with limited awareness of the world and the need for 24-hour care, without physically being close to death.

"Comfort care," which is the soft, implicit but not legally defined version of hospice, is likely to already be in place. Person-centered approaches to dementia care are essentially comfort-oriented, in many respects, already. We lack the rules and boundaries to deal with the key issues here of pain and quality of life because of our ignorance of what it is like to live with Alzheimer's and related diseases.

In "Alzheimer's Disease in Real Life—The Dementia Carer's Survey," Jim Jackson summarizes the key issues here from a medical perspective:

> Unlike these other serious illnesses, Alzheimer's disease (AD) and dementia are extremely difficult to categorize into neat stages of progression that are typically used to determine whether hospice care is appropriate. Life expectancy is difficult, if not impossible, to pinpoint for a patient affected by AD and related conditions like vascular dementia, Lewy Body dementia, and frontotemporal dementia.
>
> Furthermore, patients in the later stages are usually unable to communicate things like pain or discomfort. This means that family caregivers and even their loved ones' physicians can have a tough time deciding when to call in hospice.

We can often quickly see that someone with a terminal illness is suffering and in pain because they can describe these conditions to us, while we cannot reach the same conclusions for a person with dementia. In the early stages or midstages where communication is possible, life is inconvenienced by the illness but suffering and proximity to end of life do not meet the standards needed for hospice.

In the midstages to late stages we don't know. Suffering is evident, but it is different from pain or other forms of physical suffering because we have no standards for mental anguish. Look at our difficulty with PTSD. We can understand the trauma that war can cause in the mind, yet we dance away from giving full regard to those suffering because it is considered a mental condition.

Alzheimer's music programs have done a remarkable job of "waking" minds that appear to have been sleeping for many years in the later stages of the disease. The right music can bring joy, laughter, and other emotions—surprising many who assumed the person inside was no longer reachable. I wonder if this is enough. Is our celebration of a small victory here, reaching into the Alzheimer's mind and plucking out emotions and feelings, sufficient to say that life in this condition with compromised memory and limited functionality is a quality life or a life without pain and suffering? Do you want this life? Probably not.

Music is offering one important dimension of comfort care. We have reached deep into a consciousness that was assumed to be asleep and pulled out some strong emotions. But we have not been able to judge the depth of the pain and suffering.

And for the most important question here—if we can reach into these "locked" minds with music and pull out meaningful responses (the emotions experienced in hearing the music), can we reach in using other tools and get to the fundamental issues related to life and pain and suffering? Can we find a way to ask about death in this context or if the pain and suffering encourages speeding death for any reason? I don't know the answer. If it was possible for you say "stop, I have reached my limit of pain and suffering," would you want to communicate this to your caregivers? If we could create a Red Button to help here, would you want to use it?

11

Why Are People with Dementia Denied Hospice Care?

People with dementia are not denied hospice care, but because we don't understand how to quantify the life expectancy of someone living with dementia or the degree of the pain and suffering they are experiencing, we make access to hospice for them quite difficult.

Many of the issues that currently block people with dementia from receiving hospice care were summarized in the previous chapter. The two core problems here are these:

1. Someone—a family member, a physician, treatment staff or another qualified person—has to make a determination that the person with dementia will likely die in the next six months. For the reasons described, these are tough decisions.

2. Because our understanding of pain and suffering with dementia is so limited, family and professionals involved are reluctant to use these concepts as a criteria for initiating hospice, even when medical directives or a conversation with the patient make it clear that life quality has descended to an unacceptable level.

Because dementia itself is rarely the cause of death, hospice decisions are complicated. While there are many peaceful, natural deaths for people living with dementia, *because the cause of death in most cases is not dementia but some other condition* such as a stroke, cancer, severe urinary tract infections, pneumonia, or many other diseases that can end life, many other deaths are not peaceful or benign and can involve considerable pain and suffering for the individual and their families.

Given this context, the stated goal of hospice for people with dementia is relevant and appropriate here (quoted from a blog at The Alzheimer's Reading Room):

> Palliative care for a person with dementia is defined as "aggressive symptom management for maximum quality of life at the present time." The goal is to treat and remove, or reduce, symptoms that are bothering the person who is deeply forgetful. Symptoms such as pain, or problems like urinary tract infections, are handled in ways that make sense to the person living in Alzheimer's World.

Palliative care in most cases represents hospice; this is where, for a person with dementia, things become complicated and choices vanish. Consider these alarming statistics. While it is estimated that 60 to 70 percent of people with dementia would benefit from hospice at the end of their life, *only 10 percent actually receive hospice care*, despite the good intentions of caregivers, physicians, and others involved.

Why? As we saw in the previous chapter, it is complicated.

- The individual with dementia cannot choose hospice because hospice requires that the individual be judged "mentally competent" to make this decision. It is extremely rare for a person with dementia to meet this requirement in a late stage.
- In the case of dementia, there are exceptions to the traditional hospice requirements and the "mentally competent" rule can be overlooked in most cases, placing the burden of the decision on the medical staff and caregivers.
- Most of the time, however, family, caregivers, and physicians are reluctant to make the call that the individual has less than six months to live. The result is that hospice is not started. While some form of palliative care may be started near the end of life, this is not guaranteed (in fact, many caregivers I interviewed would fight to prevent this because it acknowledges the start of an inevitable slide toward death).

- The conclusion: many people with dementia undergo unnecessary pain and suffering before their death because caregivers and medical staff are reluctant to make the judgment that hospice is necessary now—and because few people understand the concept of pain and suffering with dementia.

At the conclusion of a recent workshop on hospice presented to individuals in a local retirement center, I asked the presenters about how pain and suffering would be defined for people with dementia. The answer shocked me, but to anyone living with Alzheimer's, it is probably not surprising:

> We treat people with dementia just like people without dementia. We judge their health based on their medical status and their general well-being, not their mental status. Being forgetful, even to the point of not knowing family or being able to function with daily routines, is not a basis for hospice. Most of these people, with their memory no longer working, are passive and content. We would not define this as pain and suffering.

This is a big part of the problem. Ask a person in the early stages of dementia about this conversation or ask yourself. At what point, when the mind and memory disconnect from the world, your family and friends, your daily routines and the things that bring relevance and joy to your life, are you considered to be suffering? Or is this a border that you will never reach?

What I have learned is that most people with dementia do have boundaries here and that living in a semivegetative state is not acceptable—not just because they are helpless and not engaged with the world but also because of the burden this presents to their caregivers, family budgets, and many other factors.

Many of these people with dementia would like to say, “When these conditions occur, regardless of my physical health, it is time to begin considering my death because I am in pain and I am suffering—even if the medical community cannot acknowledge this. I want a choice here. I want to find a way for my voice to be heard even though I cannot speak. I want to stop the train when these circumstances occur. I want a Red Button.”

12

Assisted Death and Suicide

Suicide is not common for people living with dementia, and assisted deaths are also rare, except perhaps in the context of a hospice program where denial of treatment speeds death.

Suicide is not common for people living with dementia, but it does occur and does so most frequently during the early stages of the disease's progression. The diagnosis of Alzheimer's, especially for people younger than 80, can be devastating. That's why many physicians, the Alzheimer's Association, and society, which promotes the stigma, pile on woes with fear, a helpless attitude (since there is no cure), and misperceptions.

When you add to this the anxiety, the financial stress, and the uncertainty this news brings to families and relationships, the pile of woes just grows that much higher. Despite all of these negative factors, it is estimated that less than 3 percent of people with an Alzheimer's diagnosis will take their own life within the first two years; and after this time the odds are much lower.

Suicide, of course, is one of the few Red Buttons that a person living with dementia has the opportunity to control. Probably it would be more common if the average age of onset was younger, but that is not the case. The other important option is the broad class of aid-in-dying provisions that are gradually becoming more common across the country as state legislatures make them legal and available. Often described as laws to insure "death with dignity," euthanasia and assisted deaths are the most common forms of aid-in-dying. They are accessible as Red Buttons for anyone living with constant pain, a terminal illness, or other conditions as long as the individual is judged to be mentally competent.

In the case of dementia, however, the issues are much the same as for hospice care but more restrictive. If, during a healthy stage of your life, you set up the requirements for a Red Button when life quality was diminished to a specific degree and requested an assisted death at this time, it is very unlikely your request would be honored if you had dementia. There are many issues here, not the least of which is our understanding of pain and suffering in this context.

In states like Colorado, California, New Jersey, and Washington where strong aid-in-dying options exist for people, a disappointing countertrend is quietly emerging to erode these important rights. Hospital systems across the country have been in the process of consolidating for many years, with the result that only ten major systems are still operating today and five of these are Catholic mixed with other faith-based organizations. Their core belief—that patients experiencing suffering that cannot be alleviated should be helped to appreciate the Christian understanding of redemptive suffering—means that healthcare providers in these systems "may never condone or participate in euthanasia assisted suicide in any way."

Despite the issues associated with hospice and dementia described in the last two chapters, hospice offers the best alternate form of assisted death through its focus on comfort rather than extending life. If an individual with dementia is nearing the end of life and it is obvious to everyone involved that they are suffering, decisions made to provide comfort versus extending life can directly or indirectly lead to death—or at least speed death. Obviously, the idea of death with dignity is a complex issue on many dimensions here.

The heart of the problem comes down to two key questions for family and care professionals:

1. If an individual's medical directives or Conversation (discussed in chapter 18) make it clear that when their life quality (defined by specific mental and physical conditions) reaches a specific threshold in which they want to speed the process of death, are we willing to honor this request?

2. Are we willing to expand our traditional understanding of pain and suffering to include dementia-related conditions?

13

The Vessel and the Spirit

Death is often the story of a gradual physical decline ending when one or more of the body's essential support systems fails and life ends naturally. This is the story of the vessel. What about the spirit? The presence of the spirit during life and especially at the end of life is as strong and relevant as our treatment of the vessel. A common observation from professionals and family is that the person was ready, had a sense of when it was time to die, and made this transition peacefully and without anxiety.

The traditional path from life to death is often the story of a gradual physical decline ending when one or more of the body's essential support systems fails; life ends naturally or with the blessing of comfort care intended to reduce pain and suffering and eliminate unnecessary life-extending treatments. Hidden within this traditional description, however, is much of the magic that endows life and the essence of every person with their uniqueness as humans on this planet and the divine mysteries we cannot comprehend. There is the vessel, of course, which is failing; but also, not to be forgotten, is the spirit.

When we speak of physical death and also of the pain and suffering that leads to death, often we are referring to properties of this physical shell that we have inhabited for our time on earth. Throughout 2017 and 2018 we witnessed the demise of one of our country's great heroes, John McCain, who was suffering from terminal brain cancer. His body slowly deteriorated until eventually all means of support were stopped and the body's physical systems were allowed to finally fail. End of the story.

Well, not quite. Was there any point during this period that we witnessed his spirit failing? I don't think so. In fact, as the events of his life were replayed many times on the media, we could see that even in the darkest hours, his spirit shone with an uncommon brilliance, illuminating his integrity and courage for all to witness. Was there any doubt that he took this light and the spirit it represents with him until his final breath? I don't think so.

All end-of-life stories are tales about these two themes, the eventual failure of the vessel and the separate adventures of the spirit. They don't all end as happily or dramatically as John McCain's life story. Both the vessel and the spirit can suffer and fail in many ways, but often the story of the spirit is unique and not tied to the body's demise. My parents both maintained the fullness of life and joy in their spirits until the moment of their physical death even though their physical shells were battered by the inconveniences of aging—Dad struggled to walk and breathe while Mom was legally blind.

Many others, especially those who are fortunate enough to follow the path of good death described in chapter 5, are blessed in this way. The physical shell declines through normal aging processes and disease, but the spirit prevails.

What happens with dementia and other disorders that take away full conscious awareness of our shared reality and distort our memories? We can see the decline in the vessel (which can be very limited), yet the challenges faced by the spirit are often much less transparent. With Alzheimer's, for example, the connections that tie logical, rational parts of the spirit to this world may have been diminished to such a degree that we, as observers and caregivers, no longer understand. There is no speech coming that shouts messages of love, wisdom, or patriotism. But does this matter? Is the spirit less important because it no longer shares our common reality? What if John McCain could not speak but gave hand signals to communicate? Would this change how we viewed him or his death?

This topic is one of the great conundrums associated with dementia and other afflictions that impact mental functioning—and also the source of much of the stigma. As the vessel suffers and declines with aging, we typically make no assumptions about the spirit and the person being diminished. Damage to the vessel is understood and accepted. It is a normal part of aging. Damage to the mind and the spirit and to consciousness—that is different. Here is where our understanding (and our level of comfort) ends.

Now the role of the Red Button becomes more evident. The button is about the choice to end the suffering that the vessel must endure, yet at the same time it is clearly an extension or manifestation of the spirit. Ultimately, it is not the physical suffering that matters here but how the spirit interprets and tolerates this suffering that guides our choices. Because dementia-related hospice decisions are collective choices based on historical videos or documents, the spirit is still strong and focused, but it is the collective will and spirit of family, friends, and other caregivers that will decide. This is why a video is so important to support tough choices. Watching a family member speak directly on video is engaging the spirit and the intentionality of that spirit. Watching the decline of a person no longer communicating engages only a limited shell of the full being.

Every caregiver who has immersed themselves in the life of a companion with dementia understands the importance and beauty of this collective spirit. We are not alone and have never been alone, but our egos often mask this fact with our goals, achievements, and self-driven life. The step that a friend or family member takes in going from *caring from MY perspective,* where the task of caregiving is often viewed as a time-consuming inconvenience, to *caring from OUR perspective*, which embraces the collective spirit, is huge—but many loving caregivers, dealing with many kinds of illness or just aging, willingly take this step.

Dementia can hasten this process because every precious moment lived openly, with love and without evaluation, opens the door to the universe of spirit. Not everyone is prepared or willing to relinquish their ego's demands in order to provide the empathy and understanding needed to be a great care partner for a person living with dementia, but when this happens, the now-shared spirit makes a Red Button possible.

14

The Dementia Train

Your journey on the dementia train is a journey few others will understand because they have imposed their version of reality on you and do not grasp the essence of your world. It is a journey that will last until your eventual death.

The story of the dementia train is in many ways similar to Sartre's *No Exit*. Once you are on the train, your reality becomes that of the collective perception of others and their view of dementia. You are locked into this reality for eternity or death. There is no way, currently, for you to get off the dementia train if you choose to do so. There is no STOP button to push or conductor who can hear your requests. Your reality is the artificial reality imposed by others. That is why the idea of a Red Button does not exist except in limited ways. But what if it did? Stretch your imagination for a moment and consider how this might work.

The dementia train is a bit like the train Harry Potter used for his annual trips to Hogwarts. It has an entrance that no normal person (the muggles or a nondementia population) can see. Once you are traveling on the train, you are invisible to the normal world, which only sees your shadow through the filters imposed by a dementia diagnosis.

If you need help from the conventional world, you are not likely to get it, because this world cannot understand you except using *dementia-speak*, a language you hate because it is both demeaning and limited. Is this sounding familiar? Living with dementia, you understand these concepts well. You can also now see the great dilemma presented by the idea of a Red Button.

You may very well know, in your mind and in your world, that it is time to get off the train of life, but how are you going to do this when in conventional earth-reality you don't exist? Imagine in Harry Potter's case that, to the muggles, his train represented no more than mysterious shadows that passed through the landscape. How are you going to pull a message from weird moving shadows? We have been waiting many years for a person who has been living in the world inhabited by those with late-stage Alzheimer's to return and give us the details on their journey, but this has not happened.

The Red Button represents an important slice of reality in the real world, not the dementia world. But how do you gain access when pushing it on the train, begging for it to stop, means something completely different to the muggles, who are standing by the tracks observing? How can you tell them you are suffering? Could a medical directive or video from the past be enough here? Perhaps, but only if they are listening carefully and are willing to act with firmness and courage at the crucial time.

15

It's About Pain and Suffering

The concepts of pain and suffering are clearly concrete when they apply to conditions such as continuous, ongoing pain from a terminal illness or severe injuries. However, what about mental anguish, frustration, repetitive behaviors, loss of short-term memory, and other dementia-related conditions so frightening they terrify families the moment a diagnosis is made? Do these constitute pain and suffering?

The classic definitions of pain and suffering are easily understood to apply to conditions such as continuous, ongoing pain from a terminal illness or severe injuries, or the inability to eat or breathe independently, or other extreme circumstances where an individual is consciously hurting or suffering in a manner we can all relate to in some form. Decisions about assisted death or hospice are often "less gray" when one of these situations applies.

Often adding to clarity here (which can make these decisions less contentious) is age. Concepts such as comfort care, hospice, or even assisted death are a common part of aging now, so the threshold for pain and suffering may be easier to cross if you are older and nearer the point where a natural death would be expected.

Elderly or not, our understanding of pain and suffering is much clearer when it is connected with diseases or physical conditions that, to any observer, obviously involve pain and suffering. In this context, when there is no cure or long-term resolution available for the problem, the idea of comfort care or assisted death can be offered with few religious or moral conflicts because it represents mercy in a form that we expect and understand. Pain and suffering associated with a terminal illness is the classic situation here that sets up the opportunity for hospice or other forms of comfort care today.

Family decisions about hospice are often not easy to make because they involve an acknowledgment that death is imminent and that by providing maximum comfort you will shorten the life of a loved one. It is fortunate that in many cases, however, the person impacted by the decision is mentally sound and can have a voice. Even when this is not true, when the form of pain and suffering is obvious, and both the personal and medical community can agree to offer mercy or respite from the suffering—some form of comfort care is the result.

People living with dementia have a more complicated path here and fewer options because, in general, our normal definitions of pain and suffering do not apply to the midstages and late stages of dementia unless other health conditions are also present. Their boundaries are not likely to be respected by healthcare providers and many others for two important reasons: (1) Pain and suffering is not well understood in the context of living with dementia; and (2) While the condition is terminal, it may very well be terminal in two or three or five years, not a few weeks or months.

Some of the guidelines applied to people with dementia for a hospice decision include these:

- Constant, elevated levels of stress and anxiety
- Complete dependence on others for assistance with everyday activities (such as eating, bathing, and toileting)
- The inability to walk without assistance
- The inability to speak, with only a few intelligible words and phrases available

Remember, however, that in part because of these guidelines, only 10 to 11 percent of people with dementia (as the primary diagnosis) are given access to hospice. An unfortunate but common path to death, without hospice, starts with an infection followed by urinary and fecal incontinence, difficulty swallowing and breathing, and a weakened immune system.

At some point a hospital stay will become necessary and, caught in the powerful, end-of-life interventions that are available to physicians today (such as short-term medications with side effects or feeding tubes or breathing support), the choice to die quietly with a focus on comfort is lost. Hospitals and physicians respect life, so it is normal for them to go to great lengths to save a life; but once this process is started, it is easy for quality-of-life considerations for the individual to be lost in the battle. You will need a strong advocate to stay the course once your path has deviated in this direction.

Let me ask you a difficult question. Which condition is more deserving of the mercy associated with hospice care: living with terminal lung cancer with no hope of improvement and suffering from constant pain, or living with advanced Alzheimer's, with no hope of improvement, and suffering from a complete mental breakdown with limited awareness of the world and no recognition of daily routines or the people in your life? Obviously, there is no easy answer to this question; it is also obvious that both conditions deserve our consideration. In the case of cancer, we confront the pain and surrounding circumstances directly with many forms of help and choices. In the case of Alzheimer's, we mostly look away, our decision confounded by the individual's inability to tell us of their pain and suffering.

To keep your choice for a dignified ending open as hospice becomes appropriate, you must set up the Red Button or conditions about a hospice decision earlier, while you are healthy. Remember that hospitalization is about fixing the physical body, while hospice is about nurturing the patient's whole person, physically, emotionally, spiritually, and mentally.

Part III

Creating Your Red Button

16

Good Choices Begin with Positive Self-Talk

What we say to ourselves, not others, provides the direction and intentionality that drive all important choices. This running conversation, taking place continually in most minds, is called self-talk. It is the key to making good decisions about life and death.

What we say to ourselves, not others, provides the direction and intentionality that drive all important choices. This running conversation, taking place continually in most minds, is called self-talk. In these conversations there is a "talker," generating the words that are spoken silently, and there is a "listener" somewhere in our mind "hearing" these spoken words. Often the talker is associated with the left brain and the speech center of the cerebral cortex, and the listener is linked to the wholistic, image-oriented right brain, but probably this explanation is too simplistic.

Choices about which dessert to order, which TV show to watch, or whether to go shopping today or visit the gym can often be made quickly and intuitively without much conscious thought or self-talk. Important choices about jobs, relationships, giving, and certainly end-of-life decisions (and the other topics in this book) can, however, be challenging for a number of reasons.

Mention "my death" or "Alzheimer's" or "cancer" or "divorce" in a conversation and you may notice that while your speech sounds normal, underneath there is a catch, a sigh, an emotional hit or self-talk that is negative and fearful. This is part of the reason conversations about death are so difficult. To have a conversation with another person we also, internally, are carrying on a parallel conversation with ourselves.

Before you can make good choices about the end of life and communicate these choices to family and friends, your self-talk about these topics needs to be positive and future-oriented; otherwise, your own fear and hesitation may trigger their fear and natural reluctance to talk about these subjects through a process called mirroring.

How do you do this? It's remarkably easy and almost foolproof. You create a set of five to six affirmations or positive statements about the end-of-life topics in this book that are most important and read them aloud a couple of times a day. The positive choices will begin to guide your thinking and conversations with others. It is a bit like learning to swim or overcoming any other obstacles in life. As you tackle them, step-by-step, they become more familiar and less fearful. The hit inside that comes from talking about death (your death or that of someone close to you) diminishes as you repeat the affirmations, and others will sense this change in you as well.

Here are some examples of affirmations:

- Death is a natural part of the process of living.
- Love continues forever.
- I am ready to let go of my fear of death.
- I accept the gift of this day joyfully and will live it fully.
- My actions today, preparing for my eventual death, will be gifts for my loved ones when I am gone.
- Conversations about death allow me to accept and embrace this stage of life without fear.
- I release all fear and doubt to embrace the infinite.
- I know that I am loved now and will be forever.

17

Create a Will and Medical Directives

The Red Button is about choices at the end of life and this includes the option to terminate life under certain conditions. Your medical directives are the first line of defense here and offer legal, widely accepted options for ending life when the circumstances demand it.

Most important conversations about death begin with the basic legal and medical documents that you will prepare as a routine part of creating a will. One of these documents—your medical directive or advanced healthcare directive, completed routinely as part of the package—directly addresses some core issues linked to the Red Button. It is a legal document in which a person specifies what actions should be taken for their health if they are no longer able to make decisions for themselves because of illness or incapacity. Since some of these actions lead to death to reduce pain and suffering, the document can form the heart of your Red Button when you are unable to choose.

A broader and more powerful form of medical directive is called the Five Wishes (a program of Aging with Dignity, www.fivewishes.org):

- Wish 1: Assigning a healthcare agent or person you want to make your care decisions when you cannot.
- Wish 2: Creating a living will and defining what life support and other medical treatments mean to you and when you would or would not want to use them.
- Wish 3: Defining comfort care that specifies what type of pain management you would like, personal grooming and bathing instructions, and options for hospice care.
- Wish 4: Specifying personal matters such as how you want people to treat you, whether you want to be at home, and religious decisions.
- Wish 5: Communicating with your loved ones what you want them to know, matters of forgiveness and remembrance, and your memorial plans.

Completing the Five Wishes booklet is a huge step toward creating a Red Button because it defines many of the core details and, in a friendly way, begins the conversations about death with your family, your attorney, and your minister. Let's be clear here. Decisions not to resuscitate or not to use a feeding tube under certain conditions are important, crucial examples of Red Buttons that you have available now.

While the basic Fish Wishes documents are excellent, there are two areas that need expansion to cover the experiences and requirements of people with dementia. One concerns the instructions to caregivers. The other describes conditions associated with starting or continuing life support.

Here are suggested additions to the Five Wishes documents to cover people with dementia.

What You Should Keep in Mind as My Caregiver:

1. Although I may not be able to speak clearly to express my feelings and needs with words or may experience other difficulties using speech to communicate, please do not think that I am no longer present or interested in communicating with you. *Please find another way to listen to me and by observing my actions, the context for the communication, and my words to understand what I am trying to say.*

2. If I am anxious, frustrated, or acting out in an inappropriate manner, there is a good chance that I am trying to communicate something to you that you are not understanding. Please try to listen, not to my words, but to what I am intending to communicate. Please view my frustration as a signal that something important is not being understood

correctly, not as an attack on you or a lack of appreciation for your help.

Other Conditions Associated with Dementia in Which I Do Not Wish to Be Kept Alive:

1. If I am experiencing the symptoms of severe cognitive decline, memory loss, and other forms of mental impairment common to the advanced stages of dementia. These symptoms include not recognizing family and friends; experiencing repetitive behaviors most of the time; being stuck in passive, nonresponsive states most of the time; being frustrated and angry most of the time; and others.

2. If my cognitive functioning has declined to the point that I am unable to complete everyday activities such as using the toilet, bathing, dressing, or feeding myself.

3. If my behavior, my speech, my emotionality (or lack thereof), the absence of joyful moments, and/or other conditions suggest I am experiencing constant mental pain and suffering.

Note that both of these programs initiate conversations about death with your family in a familiar, benign manner since they are so widely accepted. These first conversations pave the way for giving you choices in the new territory that death with dementia and pain and suffering with dementia represent. Have them as soon as possible and move on to the tougher conversations described in the chapters that follow.

18

Have the Conversation

It can be difficult for family and friends to honor your choices at the end of your life because your wishes may run counter to the medical establishment's goal of extending life, by whatever means, for as long as possible. In these circumstances it will be tough for them to "pull the plug" as you have requested in your medical directives. Having the Conversation can help here.

The Conversation Project is a public engagement initiative (stimulated in part by Atul Gawande's book, *Being Mortal*) with the goal of transforming the physician-patient relationship near the end of life by having every person's wishes for end-of-life care expressed and respected.

The key to making this happen is to have conversations with family and friends about the way you want to live at the end of your life and the kinds of care that are appropriate. Creating your medical directives and/or completing the Five Wishes questions are huge steps for expressing your needs in this context and creating options for a Red Button, but these are not always followed by frank, open conversations with key members of your family because in our culture it is so difficult to talk about death.

A large percentage of Americans, 50 to 60 percent, do not die a good death but instead die in healthcare institutions tethered to machines and tubes at bankrupting costs. This occurs despite the fact that (based on medical directives) most would prefer to be at home, in comfort, surrounded by family. This occurs because serious illnesses near the end of life often require hospitalization to extend life, and family are reluctant to not go along. Physicians, by their nature and training, want to extend life using all of the tools available. Losing a life is considered losing the battle as a physician, despite the poor quality of life that a victory may achieve.

The Conversation Project wants to take back control here for the individual near the end of life so these key decisions about extending life are made by family and caregivers with full knowledge of what the person wanted and intended. Having conversations about death, conditions associated with the quality of life, and the Red Button are essential to ending a good life with a good death.

Since it may be difficult, when the time comes, for key family members to deny treatments that can extend life at the cost of life quality, a video version of the conversation becomes very important. In the video the person describes much of what is included in the medical directives—where they want to live, what treatments they do or do not want, and what conditions make a life unsuitable to continue.

Note that it is a luxury to be able to have these conversations near the end of life. People living with dementia and many others do not enjoy this luxury and need to have them earlier. If you have dementia, when you have completed the revised version of the Five Wishes booklet (explained in chapter 17), include dementia-related conditions in the conversation as you make the video. The challenge here is that the concept of pain and suffering for those individuals living with dementia is not well understood, so you will need to think about when, for you, these conditions represent the point where pushing the Red Button is appropriate.

The Conversation Project has created a special set of additions for people living with Alzheimer's or dementia that address quality of life issues unique to these diseases—to be included in the conversation with family. These are so useful and relevant I have included information on them below.

If you are reading this book because you or a family member or friend have dementia, I strongly recommend three actions:

1. Complete the Five Wishes questions (which will include medical directives).

2. Have conversations with your family and others about your end-of-life wishes. Use the Conversation Starter Kit on The Conversation Project website

(http://TheConversationProject.org). It is excellent. I have included questions from this kit here to share what kinds of dementia-related conditions might be relevant to you in defining life quality.

3. Do a brief video summarizing your wishes for end-of-life care based on these discussions, paying special attention to any conditions that represent a Red Button for you. When family or other caregivers need to make tough decisions near the end of your life, having your wishes and intentions expressed in your own words is particularly helpful.

Using the Conversation Starter Kit for People Living with Dementia

The Conversation team recognized quickly that many users were people with dementia and their associated families and friends, so in 2016 they created a special version of the kit to support this population. While it is similar to the original materials, there are a few important additions:

- It makes clear the importance of supporting an individual's *personhood* through the process of living with dementia.
- It offers many suggestions for how to address end-of-life issues with people in the different stages of dementia. In the early stages of the disease the standard approach works fine with some consideration given to the unique conditions that limited mental functioning creates. For people already in a

midstage to late stage of dementia, family and other caregivers represent them by collective proxy.

- It acknowledges the limitations of organizations such as the Alzheimer's Association and also physicians (who may "abandon" individuals with a dementia diagnosis, lacking a cure or other tools) and encourages people to reach out to more positive, supportive groups.
- Finally, supporting a person with dementia is about making things very concrete and clear, not abstract. Taking a conceptual approach to choices around life support or other end-of-life decisions probably won't work. Making the options clear and direct so that the decision is a yes or no works much better.

The team's final summary comment: Alzheimer's is a brain disease. Treat it like a disease. Don't treat it like a stigma. As long as you are ashamed and embarrassed about what is happening, you don't get help.

19

Tell Your Story and Leave a Legacy

Sharing your life stories and history with others creates a kind of immortality because these will persist long after you are dead. Leaving a legacy creates your presence in the lives of others that may last for many generations. A legacy is a special collection of gifts that endure.

Conversations about death and the end of life can be difficult for mortals, but for immortals they are not a problem. So why not choose immortality? What does this mean? You certainly would not choose to live forever with dementia. But what if the healthy part of your life lasted indefinitely?

It does! Stories about you and your life, your history, your experiences with family and friends who survive you—all of these will persist for years or generations after your death. Notice that in the context of this new immortality you are experiencing, death is just a natural part of the process. Your physical body will die but many other parts of you will remain, indefinitely.

Perhaps knowing this softens the idea of death and makes the discussion of end-of-life options easier. Perhaps not. In any case, intentionally choosing to take actions now that will create your presence in the lives of others after your death changes things. Death remains a definite ending for your physical being but you will be remembered for much more than this. For some, religion offers a path to eternal life and immortality; for others this is not such a sure thing, since evidence for it is limited.

Here are some simple actions you can do now that will guarantee your immortality and add quality to your life:

- Tell your stories. Write or tell your favorite stories about your life to family members so they become known and shared.
- Create a biography. While writing a full biography is likely to be more of a task than you want to undertake, just create a highlight version or an outline.
- Do an interview. Find someone in the family or hire someone to interview you and then create a version of this as a history that you can share in written form or video or audio.

In each of these cases you are accepting the inevitability of your death and leaving gifts to your family or friends that will endure. In so doing, you are quietly becoming immortal.

Making the choice to tell your story to family, friends, and future generations or to leave a legacy does something remarkable. It brings conversations about your death into a natural, comfortable place. It also suspends time, for the history of your life is timeless. It is a living part of your life now but it will persist, perhaps for many generations, after your death.

I remember many things about my grandparents, but what sticks are the stories that define their character. My grandfather on my mom's side of the family was a physician and head of health services in Hardeman County, Tennessee. For many years, remote areas of the county did not have access to a dentist, so Grandfather rigged up a dental chair in a pickup truck! Then, he would spend a day or two each month fixing cavities and pulling teeth as needed.

What are your stories that are being shared? Are they currently part of your life? Does your family have access to a written copy of your history, including information on growing up, work, where you lived, how you thought about the world, your greatest adventures, your friends, your spouse, successes and failures—and so forth? Do you have pictures or movies to share? What about articles or publications or anything you have written? Ask your children and grandchildren for help, if needed. Digital devices today can capture these kinds of information quickly and preserve it.

The concept of a legacy is another powerful affirmation of your life that suspends death for eternity. A legacy is an intentional choice about death that can impact the quality of your life now and the quality of your family's lives for eternity. With a legacy, you are saying I accept the inevitability of death and wish to leave gifts to my family that will endure.

A legacy is a gift handed down across generations. In families that are financially fortunate, a legacy can very well mean, in part, an inheritance. But most of the time a legacy refers to a broad class of material or intellectual items that are intentionally left to a specific friend or family member that have some emotional or physical value. My grandfather left me a leather case from his history in Belgium during World War I, as an example.

The story of your life or parts of your life, when written, is a powerful legacy to be passed down for generations. Articles that you have created and pass to specific family members, such as books or paintings or other possessions, become part of your legacy. Your actions in key situations at work, at home, or in wartime become part of your legacy.

Others may help to create your legacy through their stories, but your actions, especially your concrete decisions to leave things in your possession now to those who can benefit from them after your death, are just as important. Sit down now, make a list, and be sure these bequests are included in your will.

20

Make the Choices on Your Bucket List

Living deliberately and intentionally today helps to create the willpower and confidence needed to make decisions about the end of life, to create medical directives, and to have the conversation with your family. A bucket list is an excellent tool to support this process.

What does the Red Button have to do with your bucket list? It's simple. Both are choices to live intentionally and proactively. At the time a Red Button is relevant, you will need every ounce of your willpower to "push it" or communicate to others to push it. Living with a bucket list, at any age or in any condition, is living forward with an interest in and focus on those things that bring quality to your life. A bucket list is a light but powerful version of "Make A Wish." You are choosing to postpone death by living. It is as simple as that.

How do you use a bucket list? Here are the steps:

1. Make your list by selecting five to ten activities you would like to do before you die. If you are young and healthy and affluent, your options are unlimited. If you are restricted because of age or health or finances, more immediate, local options will work fine. What's on your list does not matter as long as it is possible for you to live it.

2. Post your list on your door or desk or another place that you see every day.

3. Select each item on the list and with the help of family or friends (if needed) plan how you will experience it and then do it. Traveling to Tibet will take more work than an afternoon visit to the zoo, but both are great examples of bucket list items.

4. Mark the item, showing it is completed, and celebrate your accomplishment.

When you commit to doing something and then follow through, that's a powerful affirmation of life and it makes other choices, especially tough ones associated with the end of life, easier to make. With each completed item on the list, death takes a step back from the door.

21

Celebrate the End

Finish making good choices now by writing a draft obituary. Make it a celebration of the items you want remembered by others. Remember, it is not about death but about what matters in your life now.

Every New Year I repeat an exercise that to many seems bizarre yet for me helps to ground everything I do in the months that follow. I spend an hour writing a brief, one-page obituary. Then I look back over the previous year to see how much of it is true and how I want to use it for guidance in the current year.

An obituary, created in the present moment, is less about death (although some day that will not be true) than it is about reflection on what matters. Was he a character, a good friend, a good father, or a good spouse? Was he timid or fearless? What did he stand for? How are people celebrating his life, his work, his accomplishments and his follies?

The Red Button is about living and dying on your own terms. It is about choosing the conditions that may surround the end of your life. Your obituary, at the end, is a celebration of your life and how you want to be remembered. Your obituary today is a statement about how you want to live and what you would like others to remember about you.

Here is a simple exercise that makes conversations about your death much easier and more positive. Note that you can also be leading this exercise as part of a process to help a loved one.

1. Write a brief, one-page obituary. Think of it as a story, not necessarily a documentary. What would make your heart fill with joy if others described you in this way?

2. Begin to make the obit part of your life by living the story. Let it become part of your everyday self-talk.

3. Enjoy the power and sense of fulfillment that comes from living even a small part of the intentions expressed in your obit.

A great obituary is always part real, part fiction. Let your exercise here tap into the deep power and peace that comes from linking your life now with stories that will cross over into eternity.

Part IV

Using the Red Button

22

Loving Caregiving and the Red Button

For a variety of reasons, not every person with dementia and not every dementia caregiver believes that a Red Button is necessary. They find that the process of caring for a person with dementia (or being cared for) is a meaningful, rewarding process that does not need to be terminated early.

Over the past several months as I have shared drafts of this book with friends and editors, some strong, contrary ideas about the concept of a Red Button were expressed. Two of these viewpoints are so important I wanted to include them here.

View from People Living with Dementia

Six wise friends living with dementia shared roughly the same thoughts when asked about the idea of the Red Button. "Don't talk with me about a Red Button because my choices for care and death are already stated clearly in my medical directives. If I don't want you to extend care under some circumstances, I have already expressed this clearly. No Red Button is needed to reinforce my requests or take any new actions. Enough said."

In following up I learned that this group of friends felt like they had planned for the contingencies here that mattered to them and didn't want someone else meddling at this point. None objected to the concept of having a Red Button, just to the potential of this idea to change what was already defined and in place.

View from Caregivers and Professionals

My caregiver friends, some professional and some who served as primary caregivers for a family member with Alzheimer's, had a slightly different view about why the Red Button might not be needed.

They all described how difficult this experience was, on the one hand, yet how rewarding it was to support these individuals and be present for them when needed. The dementia professionals described the love and kindness exchanged between the individuals with Alzheimer's and their primary caregivers. The point they were making to me was that, despite their loved one having dementia, life was okay and filled with many good things. It was not a life that needed ending because of pain and suffering.

The strong message here for me, as the author of *The Red Button,* is that my abstract and general definition of pain and suffering will not always apply. Many people in late-stage dementia are not experiencing pain and suffering but just a gradually diminishing lifestyle surrounded by people who care.

I think both groups have relevant points. If you already set up medical directives, then there is a good chance you have already expressed your opinions about the option of having a Red Button in some form. If a dedicated caregiver is present, with the patience and energy to persist with love, grace, and support through the later stages of dementia, that in itself is a huge blessing and definitely a kind of hospice. My father-in-law recently died under these circumstances.

At the same time, I also recognize that the majority of people in the later stages of dementia do not have a dedicated caregiver or the resources to enjoy a quiet, extended death under the watchful eye of a loving family member or other person. Their situation comes closer to that of the individuals living with dementia in 110 publicly funded homes in England for the elderly with Alzheimer's. Research on this group by a team from Oxford showed that, on average, each person received less than five minutes daily of individual attention. This is not an example of the loving care we would hope is happening, but it is also not uncommon in the United States or globally. We simply do not have the people resources or financial resources to avoid a good deal of pain and suffering in many cases.

The two points made by my friends are valid ones, nevertheless; and we will be aware that in some circumstances, for some people, the Red Button is not a real option.

23

Honoring Choices for a Red Button

There are good reasons to find the process of dying to be especially undesirable for those living with many kinds of dementias, as well as other diseases that impact mental functioning. The process can last years. The stigmas are strong. The person can be physically alive but be living in a vegetative state. Choices around palliative care are not available.

The origin of *The Red Button* is my work with the dementia community and my recent book, *Don't Rain on My Parade: Living a Full Life with Alzheimer's and Dementia.* The book originally had a chapter that discussed options for death for people living with Alzheimer's. It was an important chapter because much of the fear and negativity about Alzheimer's (promoted by the Alzheimer's Association as part of its fundraising strategy) that blocks "living fully" comes from horror stories about life and eventual death during the later stages.

After my reviewers, several of whom are living with dementia, suggested the chapter was stretching to cover a very important topic too superficially, I elected to remove it and write this short book.

There is good reason to find the process of dying to be especially undesirable for those living with many kinds of dementias as well as other diseases that impact the mind. Some of the more negative features are these:

- The process can last years.
- The person with dementia can be "alive" but have limited cognitive and physical functioning in a vegetative state.
- Choices around palliative or comfort care that can lead to a good death versus prolonging a life that is difficult are not available in most cases.
- Caregivers often pay a huge personal and, in many cases, financial price for facilitating the extended death.

Most important here, the key choice for the individual with dementia—the choice to say "uncle," I have suffered enough—is not available. There is no Red Button to push to end the suffering or let others know that you want to end the suffering. And even if this were possible, and you did have a button to push, depending on family attitudes and where you live, your decision to end your life may not be honored for legal, religious, medical, or personal reasons.

Does this sound complicated? Definitely. But can we do something that adds compassion and a degree of control to dementia-based deaths and similar situations? Probably. That is the heart of the concept of *The Red Button*.

In previous chapters I've discussed many topics connected with good deaths, ones that involved a minimum of suffering and some degree of choice for the individual. Barbara Bush, the former first lady, died in 2018. She lived a full life, was relatively healthy as she aged, was loved by many family and friends, and, as her medical condition became more marginal, requiring major, intrusive treatment options for a brief extension of life, she was able to consciously choose comfort care and die a natural death with family present.

Contrast her death with that of many people with dementia. Although it may seem extremely benign because it is so common in the deaths of many elderly people, Barbara as well as my dad had the choice to push the Red Button and consciously say, "I am ready to go." For most types of dementia, this choice is not available because, early in the dementia process, physicians, family members, care facilities—and other people and organizations that provide support—quickly and often unconsciously buy into dementia's stigma, that the person involved is no longer mentally competent.

Last year, a dear friend and neighbor living with Alzheimer's took his own life because he could see the path ahead and knew that soon he would not be able to make a choice. This is certainly one option, to push the Red Button early, while you still can. In his case, from the outside this was unfortunate, because he had many or at least several years of pretty normal living available to him. But from the outside we cannot see the fears and concerns, especially the concern over losing the ability to make a choice, that he was experiencing.

Can we do better here? For someone living with dementia, are we able to honor their choices about the quality of life made while they are still functioning well? Is there an option to have a Red Button after this threshold is passed? Can we find a way to reduce our own fears and concerns about death that make it taboo to discuss and see it as a natural and joyful part of living, anchored in the past, present, and future?

Visit your own death here for a moment. Would you choose to live an extra five years, in a comfortable but largely vegetative state, or die? Would it change your decision if you knew your family would experience many hardships during the five years, and the legacy of your life, the history you will pass on and how you will be remembered in the future, will become tainted by your death? These are tough questions that confront many people in many kinds of deaths.

24

Communication to Support a Red Button

There are three important kinds of communication that an individual with late-stage dementia can use to send messages to caregivers: emotions, recognition of something familiar, and the reporting of an internal event.

Having a Red Button is simply about owning a way to communicate your pain and suffering with dementia to others. Pushing the Red Button is sending the message that the pain and suffering is too great to want to continue living. We already understand how difficult it is to send such messages because they are often compromised by the disease's impact on communication. So what do you do? Can it be possible to communicate something as important as your suffering and as profound as your wish to choose death over continuing to live with this pain?

To begin, let's briefly examine the "messages" that we do know can come from someone living in the later stages of dementia. The types of communication fall into three categories:

1. **Emotions:** These can range from the frustration or anger that is common with dementia to contentment to the joy that music and other stimuli can produce. A wide range of emotional responses is common for most people.

2. **Recognition of something familiar:** A person, a place, a favorite object, a tool, a flower, certain foods, and many other specific items can all provoke a response indicating recognition and familiarity, with or without an associated emotion.

3. **Reporting an internal event:** Attempts to communicate a thought, a feeling, a need, an experienced memory, or other information are common but often unclear because the message is more tied to the situation than to the specific words being said. What is clear is that the communication is intended to convey some idea, memory, or need.

If we think about these communications in the context of the Red Button, we need to ask this: would we trust any of these messages to tell us that the button had been pushed, that the pain being experienced was too much? Could an emotion ever be strong enough or persistent enough to get our attention? Continued passivity without emotion and reactivity to events in the world is common, but is it enough? What about recognition? Suppose that a certain object, a stuffed animal for example, was associated with the Red Button for many years. Would we trust a specific, trained response to this object as an indication that the button had been pushed?

The same question applies to the reporting of an internal state. If we rehearsed a link between the memory of this state and the Red Button, would we honor this link as an indicator of "too much" suffering when the time came? These are tough questions and they make it clear that using a Red Button is a two-way problem: (1) The individual with dementia has to send clear communication from the fog of dementia about their wishes; (2) The family or caregiver must have sufficient confidence in this communication to take some very significant actions to promote hospice or, more likely, an assisted death.

It is easy to imagine hundreds of situations where communication of the intent to use the Red Button would not be strong or clear enough—or the will, on the caregiver's side, to interpret the message unambiguously and act accordingly is compromised by the finality of the situation or other factors. But can we think of a single situation where using the Red Button might be possible? Let's make up an example and see if it works.

Jack, age 85, has Alzheimer's and is in the sixth year after the diagnosis. In the early stages he made a video for his family expressing his wishes for an assisted death when he reached the point where he was largely passive, lacked mobility, required 24-hour care, and no longer recognized family members. He also began a daily routine where for ten minutes each morning he studied a deck of five colored cards, reading the text on each card aloud. The red, blue, green, and yellow cards all had positive text about living well during the day. The black card had a different message.

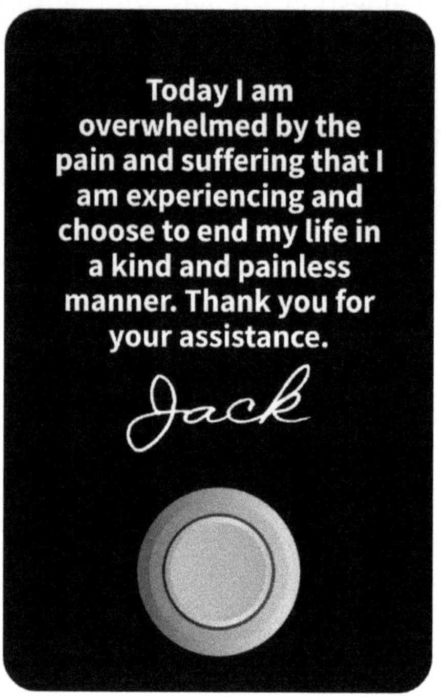

As his Alzheimer's progressed, Jack went from reading all of the cards each day to selecting one or more cards, by color, to read. Most days he chose the red card with a message about love for his family. Beginning two weeks ago, Jack's daughter Mary noticed he had selected only the black card. With her help he was able to read it aloud most days. On the fifteenth day when she asked him to select a card this is what she saw:

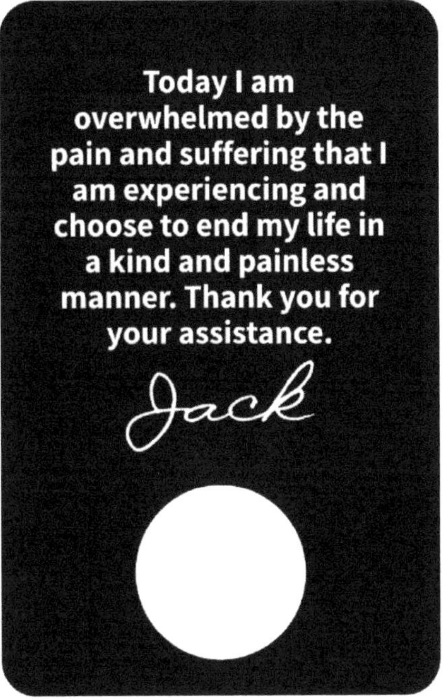

Jack had popped out the button designed as a cutout.

There are some tough questions to ask here: Would this convince you, as a family member or friend, to act? How sure are you of Jack's intent? Is there any doubt in your mind that Jack is capable of making this decision now, when otherwise he seems to be largely incapacitated? If this was not sufficient to convince you of Jack's intent, what else would it take?

In chapter 27 we look at several other options for creating and then using a Red Button.

25

Crossing the Dementia Barrier to Push the Red Button

Imagine that, for a moment, a family member or friend crossed the dementia barrier and told you they were suffering and were ready for hospice or an assisted death. This raises some interesting questions. Is this possible? Would you believe them? If so, would you be willing to act on the basis of this belief? Can a person living with Alzheimer's or another dementia push the Red Button?

Since human consciousness is dominated by our self-talk, verbal communication with others, and logical/rational thinking, it is easy to forget that the mind and our perception of reality is much more complex than this one-dimensional view. When we experience the world, we are sensing it, interpreting it, and living it on multiple dimensions of consciousness at the same time. There is the logical world but also a right-brain world of images, patterns, and wholes, a world of emotions, a world driven by shared wisdom, and other worlds that live below conscious awareness. Our minds operate within many of these worlds, some conscious, some unconscious, simultaneously.

As dementia progresses, some of these worlds or layers of consciousness are much more impacted than others. Short-term memory suffers immediately because the physical damage to the brain impacts the structures needed to consolidate what you are experiencing. Memory of specific details is also affected, but consciousness tied to broader patterns of understanding is less likely to be impacted. Concepts such as love, hero, mother, for example, are broad and likely to be maintained in some respects. Emotions and feelings are also core parts of deep consciousness.

Verbal/sequential/left-brain consciousness is the most impacted, yet the power of words as symbols that can open gateways into deeper consciousness cannot be overlooked. The word *death* can still have deeper meaning long after its abstract meaning as part of language is lost.

Intentionality is not lost as dementia progresses, but without language our filters for recognizing it in its weakened form no longer work well. This is in large part because we don't listen well. We talk, act, fumble with time when dealing with a friend who doesn't respond normally—and often this bottled up intentionality and the needs associated with them come back to us as anger and frustration.

The reality of having a Red Button is more about communication than a death wish. It is a way of expressing pain and suffering in situations where we often don't expect such communication to be possible or know how to recognize it. Acting on the basis of the alarm sounded when the Red Button is "pushed" by someone with dementia raises an entirely different set of issues. Is it possible to act to end the suffering? Are there legal, ethical, and practical solutions here?

We cannot initiate the formal hospice process, for example—it is based on a different set of criteria—because the individual's physical condition is unlikely to be terminal in the short run. Assisted death, which might be the most humane solution and fit the intentions of the person who called for help with the Red Button, may have legal or practical blocks. Ask yourself, even if your commonsense tells you that the message you are receiving from the Red Button is valid, would you be able to initiate the steps required for an assisted death?

It is important to recognize that we don't have to solve these issues for the information coming from the Red Button to be priceless. Even if you cannot act immediately to relieve the pain and suffering of a family member indicated by triggering the button, receiving the message that life is not good is a powerful incentive to not prolong life in the future when key decisions need to be made about care and medical interventions. This information also represents a profound breakthrough in our understanding of dementia in the midstages to late stages because it suggests that core parts of our human consciousness are still functioning and have always been functioning.

We, with our tendency to regard anything but verbal, logical communication as limited and compromised, have not been listening. There is an array of messages available from dementia-consciousness that we have largely missed. That is why it is so surprising to us when other layers of consciousness are stimulated by music, that a variety of complex behaviors and emotions result, reminding us that the person is very much alive.

Because the Red Button is really about communication across barriers, when we create the tools to construct a Red Button, we must also create parallel tools that support other critical messages. Consider the signal/noise problem faced by radar operators in the Arctic looking for Russian aircraft in the 1960s. Assume for a moment you were one of these operators. Which situation would you prefer?

- You are watching for a single indicator on the screen that tells you the approaching plane is Russian. Assume this indicator is correct 70 percent of the time.
- You are watching two indicators, one that identifies the plane as Russian and another that identifies the plane as "Not from the USA." Taken together, the two indicators are correct 90 percent of the time.

Obviously, this is not a tough decision. In the case of signals from dementia-reality, our confidence in the Red

Button signal is greatly increased if there are other messages available that we are also monitoring. Consider the following scenario. Our friend with dementia now has three messages they can send:

1. **The Red Button:** "Life is not good. I am in pain and suffering continually."
2. **The Yellow Button:** "Life with dementia is difficult but I am surviving."
3. **The Green Button:** "I am doing okay."

For two years the friend sent regular signals indicating the Green Button was being activated. Three months ago, they switched to the Yellow Button. Last week, the Red Button was activated. Do you think they are signaling that the pain and suffering has become intense? Probably. The reason why is that now we have different signals to discriminate among each of the three conditions, and when the Red Button signal is activated, it appears to be a deliberate, conscious act that is separate from the other messages sent. Because the individual is sending different messages, the Red Button message, when sent, has much more credibility.

Now you can understand why, in creating the following examples for constructing a Red Button, I am also recommending that you create other "buttons" or messages to use. The scenario given above is very real in that it would be wonderful if a person living in dementia-consciousness had a way to tell us that at some level they were okay. Is this possible? I don't know.

We don't currently understand the nature of dementia-reality and whether it is possible to cross the boundaries of this reality with a complex message, as suggested in the examples. Yet we do see this boundary crossed quickly with music, emotions, and responses to certain memories and even certain words. The cards I created to help with communication for late-stage dementia, the Alzheimer's Cards, can have a profound influence, stimulating communication in some cases.

With this background, here are the five paths to creating a Red Button:

1. Simple card approach
2. Wisdom concept approach
3. Pain scale approach
4. Music approach
5. Key word approach

Details on each of these approaches are offered in the next chapter.

26

The Five Paths

Simple Card Approach

Create a deck of sixteen Red Button cards using an online service such as www.makeplayingcards.com or cut out magazine images and glue them to a set of playing cards. All of the cards you create should describe how you are feeling today. For example, "I am feeling happy today." Five of the cards will describe happy, good, positive feelings; five will describe neutral or okay feelings; and five will describe negative, unhappy feelings. One card speaks about death. In my deck the colors go from bright green (positive) to yellow (neutral) to dark red (negative) for the three sets, with the death card being black with a red button. The words on the death card might read, "Today my suffering is unbearable."

Beginning in the early stages or midstages of the disease, while the individual is fully aware of the significance of the cards, each day before lunch or dinner they are given the deck and asked to describe their feelings by selecting three cards. If over a long period of time (perhaps several years) there is a progression that goes from positive/neutral to neutral/negative to negative + the death card, with the latter appearing consistently, then the sequence can be interpreted as pushing the Red Button.

Because of the familiarity of the cards and the selection process, the sequence can have a very strong meaning for the person and the caregivers. If card selection is essentially random at some point, then it does not have meaning in relationship to the Red Button; but to the degree that it appears meaningful and intentional, then it represents a strong, conscious message being sent.

Wisdom Concept Approach

Consciousness mapping systems such as the I Ching or tarot (or many others) connect with the deeper layers of consciousness by stimulating deep core concepts that underlie our existence as humans—love, mother, companionship, the folly of youth, the hero, and many others. In my example I will use tarot cards because of their spiritual power, but other systems will work just as well.

Purchase a basic deck of Rider-Waite tarot cards and separate the Major Arcana or the most powerful cards from the deck. You can use these cards directly or personalize them by substituting images of people that you know for the pictures on the card. Cards such as The Fool, The

Emperor, The Empress, The Lovers, and many others will be associated with people that you know or know of (in the case of famous individuals). Read the definitions of each card and then find a good example—or just use the cards directly.

The Fool is a special card because it represents the range of emotions and experiences in the journey through life described by the other cards. "Follow your heart" expresses the hopefulness and also the naivety of this card. On the death card (which can mean a transition where one door closes and another opens, as well as death) place a Red Button. Ultimately it will be the guide that suggests that the pain and suffering is too much.

Beginning in the early stages or midstages, while the person with dementia is fully aware and interested in creating a Red Button, you will give them the cards each day at the same time and say, "Select the card that best represents your feelings today about your past life and place it on the table." Then do the same thing for "your feelings about your life today" and "your feelings about the future." As long as possible, spend a few minutes talking about how the meaning of each card relates to the past, present, and future. The death card is as a way to represent pain and suffering experienced today or anticipated for the future.

There will be a long history of the selection of specific cards with meanings that connect with the past, present, and future. If this meaningfulness continues into late-stage dementia and the death card becomes a regular selection, the person has pushed the Red Button.

Pain Scale Approach

Begin by making a simple pain and suffering scale using my example as a guide. The scale is divided into four sections.

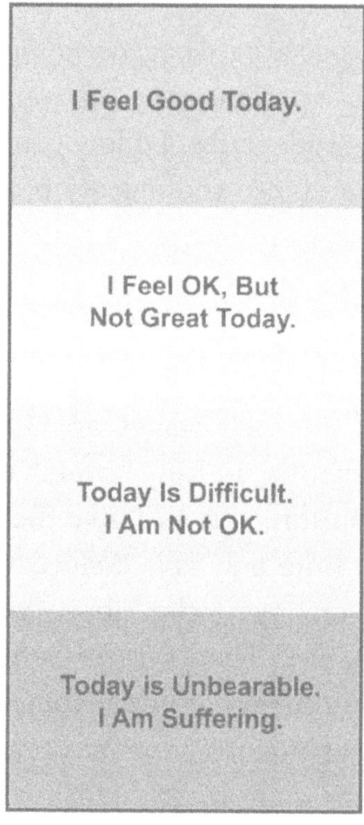

Once a day or as frequently as possible, the person with dementia and the caregiver both rate their feelings about the day by placing a coin or other marker on the scale. The results are recorded and added to a monthly chart. Selecting the red area of the scale ten days in a row represents pushing the Red Button.

This response becomes more meaningful (giving you more confidence in the interpretation) if

- The scale has been used for several years and the ratings on the red end come after a progression of more positive ratings.
- You can break a string of red ratings by creating a combination of positive events during the day that show the person is responding with some discrimination.

Music Approach

Since we know that music is a powerful emotional and cognitive stimulus through the dementia process, we might expect that it would give us a transparent window to view a potential Red Button. The procedure for using music works as follows:

1. With the help of family and friends, for someone in the early stages or midstages of dementia identify fourteen songs or short pieces of music: four that bring joy, four that are calming or quiet, four that are sad, and two that the individual would want played at their service after death.
2. Create a card with the name of the music and a picture of something that corresponds to the music (the composer, the place, the theme, for example).

3. Every day or as often as possible, starting in the early stages or midstages of dementia, have the person select one card to express how they feel today, as represented by the music. Then play this selection and one other random selection on whatever device is available. Your random selections should be from all categories, and before you play either selection remind the person of the name of the category.

4. If, over some years, there is a good sequence of selections from the positive, quiet, or sad categories that shifts to the death category for ten straight days, that is considered pushing the Red Button. If the music selected seems to correspond to the mood of the person for the day, that gives you some confidence that it is reflecting the person's inner feelings.

A variation on this approach would be to do some training in the early stages or midstages to force discrimination. Instead of letting the person select based on their feelings, you would ask them to select sad music or calm music or another category to help them associate the music with their feelings.

Key Word Approach

It has been my experience that many individuals, even in late-stage dementia, can still recognize and use words correctly and meaningfully. For this approach I recommend that you create a deck of twelve to fifteen cards, with each card containing a single word or phrase describing a feeling. Below the word or phrase will be a simple sentence explaining the meaning. The design of the cards will be similar to my Alzheimer's Communication Cards that have been used for some years as a communication device for people in the later stages.

I recommend using a range of feelings from positive to neutral to negative on the cards. The sentence below the main word or words on the card connects it with a specific feeling. For example, on the Happy Card you will see:

HAPPY
(the key word)

I am feeling **HAPPY** today.
(how it connects with the person's feelings)

The idea here is that by using the cards on a regular basis, beginning in the early stages or midstages of dementia, they will be familiar tools in the late stages when communication is difficult. The person with dementia should be shown several cards at a time and asked to select one that describes their feelings. It would be good to spread out the full set of cards, but you will need to be careful not to overwhelm the person. Going through the deck two cards at a time and selecting one of the two will generally always work, and you can use this process to gradually get to the most important card.

The Red Button card will read as follows:

The Red Button

I have pushed the Red Button
because my suffering is unbearable.

As with all previous methods, the context is very important here to demonstrate that the person is making meaningful discriminations. In this example, selecting the Red Button card five days in a row is interpreted as pushing the Red Button.

Conversations about the Red Button and creating tools to indicate that the point has been reached where pushing the Red Button is necessary can be difficult and uncomfortable. It may be easier to begin this process by using death, a process coming for all of us, as a focus for improving living today.

27

What Can We Learn from Alzheimer's Music Programs?

Music offers a potent and convincing path to communicate with people living with late-stage dementia—long after other methods have failed. There is little doubt that music can bring joy and, to a degree, wake a sleeping mind, at least briefly. What does this tell us? Can we take what has been learned from the music research and probe deeper or in ways that support additional kinds of communication?

Since hospice is often not available for people with dementia for the reasons described in this book, and the line between living-with-difficulty and living-with-great-pain is almost impossible to see when the definition is based on a mental condition, we are typically left with poor options to honor our commitments to family members suffering from a decline in mental health, regardless of the cause. Is the semivegetative state common in many cases of late-stage Alzheimer's extreme pain and suffering? Many people living with dementia said yes in my interviews for this book. Some but not all caregivers said no.

What is it like to be so disconnected from the world that your mind reboots and starts over 100 times a day, losing track of previous experiences, because of short-term memory failures? When you couple this with disassociation from the world, lack of recognition of family and friends, and failing health, is this enough to say you are in pain and suffering?

On the other hand, the music programs for people with late-stage dementia have done a remarkable job of "waking" minds that appear to have been sleeping for many years. The right music can bring joy, laughter, and other emotions—surprising many who assumed the person inside was no longer reachable. I wonder if this is enough. Is our celebration of a small victory here, reaching into the Alzheimer's mind and plucking out emotions and feelings, sufficient to say that life in this condition with compromised memory and limited functionality is a quality life or a life without pain and suffering?

Do you want this life? Probably not, but the real question is this: Once it started would you want it to continue? Music is offering one important dimension of comfort care. We have reached deep into a consciousness that was assumed to be asleep and pulled out some strong emotions. But we are not able to judge the depth of the pain and suffering.

And for the most important question here, if we can reach into these “locked” minds with music and pull out meaningful responses (the emotions experienced in hearing the music), can we reach in using other tools and get to the fundamental issues related to life and pain and suffering? Can we find a way to ask about death in this context or about the degree of pain and suffering? And what about the Red Button? If these individuals had access to a Red Button, could they push it in a way that was convincing enough for us to act on it? If I can produce joy with one kind of music or sound, can I produce an expression of pain or other emotion with other sounds? Could you be trained, before your dementia was advanced, to respond in a specific way later to sounds or words or touch or images? We don’t know.

Making Choices at the End of Life

This short book is focused on giving choices at the end of life to people living with Alzheimer's or dementia, as well as any other diseases that impact mental functioning and decision-making. If you are one of these people, your current choices are limited. You are not likely to have access to hospice care when it would be appropriate. The world does not understand the concept of pain and suffering for most mental conditions, especially the dementias. A passive, vegetative state is viewed by many as benign when compared to obvious physical pain and suffering.

The first section of this book makes it clear that the more choices you can make now, while you are healthy or in the early stages of Alzheimer's (or another disease), the better, because you may not be able to make these choices later. Having the conversation is a huge step here because video evidence of your intentions and preferences near the end of life may be necessary to overcome family resistance and the inertia of the medical community's need to keep you alive at almost any cost.

Talking about your death, leaving a legacy, creating your history, writing an obituary—all of these actions remind us of the normality of death and dying as a part of life and that to extend life beyond our physical death, in a healthy way that supports our families and friends, is very much within our means. These are easy but important choices that help to bridge now, while you are living, to the unknown of the future after your death.

One of the most important decisions your family or care partners will make is about hospice, and while hospice is granted to only 10 percent of people with dementia now, you can almost guarantee you will receive hospice, if appropriate, by setting in place the conditions to support this option today. In many respects, hospice represents your best option for an assisted death since you cannot legally make this decision on your own.

The last sections of the book have touched on many unknowns. We know, for example, that Alzheimer's and other dementias cause limited to extensive damage to the physical structure of the brain. We also know that this damage results in short-term memory loss, often leading to the breakdown of most kinds of mental/cognitive functioning, typical of the late stages of dementia. Yet because no one has returned from this late-stage condition to describe their experiences, we don't understand what is happening in the conscious and unconscious minds at this point. We know that music can spark consciousness. But what we don't know is whether this spark is a flash of lightning in a desolate landscape or a gateway into a damaged but capable mind, desperate for communication from a world that doesn't understand.

The mind in late-stage dementia is wounded, but is it absent? Is it capable of expressing pain and suffering, emotions, needs, or even intentionality? And if it can express intentionality, can it say, "Please stop my pain, I have suffered enough"?

I think the answer is yes. I think the limitations here are our limitations in the speech-oriented, nondementia reality that we all share and that the dementia mind is hungry and waiting for us to reach it with a more sophisticated, understanding approach. Music works, but it is simply a broad emotional stimulus that proves the existence of an active mind in waiting. We can do much better.

The five paths I suggest for communicating pain and suffering or the need for a Red Button are ideas grounded in my history with meditation, hypnosis, and the power of the unconscious mind. They may not work for everyone. Regardless, I have no doubt that some approach here will work and can speak directly to the healthy parts of the mind even in a late stage of dementia. My aunt, at 102, in her tenth year with Alzheimer's, did not remember me as her nephew or my cousin as her daughter but did respond joyfully to our hugs, conversations, walks, and other care.

If you are currently living with dementia, know someone living with dementia, or are a care partner or professional working to support someone with dementia, I want you (or the person with dementia) to have the choice to control your own destiny at the end of life; to express that you are in pain and suffering, or doing okay; to choose whether to start hospice, or not; and to enjoy all of the many benefits of good choices you made earlier.

The path from where you are today through the challenges that dementia will present during the next few years, until your eventual death, is not unlike a journey into a vast and unknown wilderness. You will face many challenges on your journey, but from the outside, watching those who have traveled more peacefully with less anxiety and struggle, one thing stands out: how well your care partner listens to your needs. Those individuals fortunate enough to have care partners (or better, a care partner team) intent on listening carefully to what you need, *not what you say*, have a much easier and less stressful journey.

Despite the impact that dementia will have on the cognitive areas of your mind, many other areas will be relatively unaffected—although this can vary significantly by the type of dementia. Learning to rely more on these other parts of your brain, such as the habit center, areas that support nonverbal communication, use of pattern recognition, use of emotions to communicate thoughts and needs, or learning an Alzheimer's clone language can help to support living fully and happily. None of these will solve the problems you face in your life with dementia, but they are bridges back to the world of your family and friends who are listening and want to help.

Embracing Spirit

We have a limited understanding of the spiritual plane of reality when compared with our everyday experience in the physical world. Does it even exist, based on your beliefs? Do you control it as an individual or is it part of a collective consciousness, as many believe? Does it belong to God or a religion in some way, or to everyone?

Choices about the end of life may begin with the need to reduce pain and suffering but eventually they all end in spirit. While the world will watch you suffer with dementia from the outside, without understanding your experience, it will embrace the mystery and power of your spirit. Near death, open hearts and minds will join you to fully receive the beauty of your spirit and to ignore the stigma, the struggles, and the frustrations of your journey.

My heart goes out to you as a person with dementia, a care partner, or a professional. I hope you find the ideas presented in this book to be helpful.

Acknowledgments

I want to thank the community of kind people associated with the Dementia Action Alliance who encouraged me to write this book and supported me in many ways. Thanks to the CEO, Karen Love for her helpful conversations and wisdom on this topic. Thanks to Board Chair Jackie Pinkowitz and her husband Lon who read an early draft and made a number of insightful suggestions. Thanks to Mike Belleville, one of the heroes in my last book (*Don't Rain On My Parade: Living a Full Life with Alzheimer's and Dementia*) who organized a podcast on The Red Button for a group living with dementia. Their good questions provided many valuable insights. Special thanks to Brian LeBlanc, another of my dementia heroes, who offered his ideas and shared his recent (and shocking) experiences with the medical profession and the stigma they projected. Finally, thanks to my Santa Fe friend, founder of the Alzheimer's Café, and wise counselor to people with dementia, Jytte Lokvig --- her conversations and insights always serve to ground me in the practical aspects of living with Alzheimer's.

While the topic of "living well with dementia" is alive and thriving within this community, dealing with the absence of options at the end of life, especially hospice, euthanasia and the reduction of mental pain and suffering, is much rarer and more challenging; yet, as I learned, these conversations are welcomed and badly needed. I am most grateful for the patience, support and openness offered by everyone I encountered.

Finally, I want to thank my editor, Sandra Wendel and my designer, Heidi Sutherlin. Sandra reorganized the book, giving it a much stronger focus and direction and added strength and clarity. She also guided me through the steps needed to bring it to publication. She was a kind and patient rock who kept me focused on the things that mattered. Heidi was responsible for both the excellent cover design and the book interior. She stepped me through the process of creating a good cover and was most patient with my need for many choices. I was very fortunate to have both Sandra and Heidi in my corner. Thank you!

About the Author

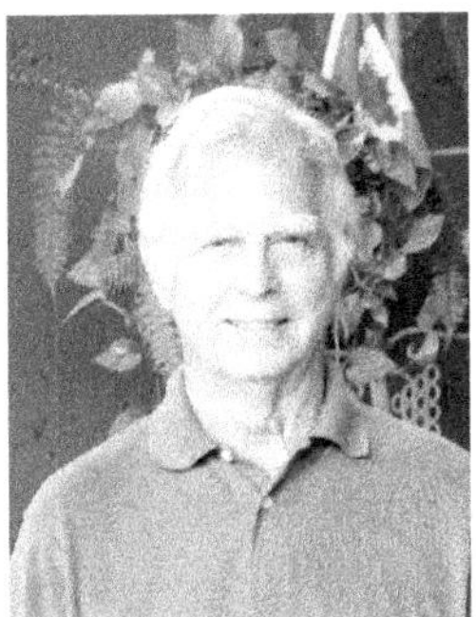

Richard Fenker is Emeritus Professor of Psychology at Texas Christian University and an author, inventor, and mathematician. He is an expert in human learning, thinking, and consciousness. His interest in Alzheimer's was sparked after interactions with his aunt Emi Lou who, while living in a late stage of the disease, was still fully conscious in many ways. The question he asked was, "What happens to human consciousness during the different stages of Alzheimer's?"

Dr. Fenker spent a year learning from dementia caregivers, people with dementia, and Alzheimer's professionals. The result was his first book on the subject, *The Long*

Moment: Communicating with the Alzheimer's Mind (2015).

For that book he invented the Alzheimer's Communication Cards (and app) to support the communication process for people in the later stages of the disease. He presented this work at the International Alzheimer's Conference in Copenhagen in 2015, where sixteen other countries requested copies of the cards (in the appropriate language, of course).

At the conference he discovered that the Alzheimer's community was rarely given any good news about the disease to support people living with dementia, to offer help in preventing it, or to suggest a cure. Of the 2,450 presentations at the conference, fewer than twenty were positive. He also learned that in the United States, the Alzheimer's Association is "big business," with most of the money raised going to salaries, the pharmaceutical industry, and research organizations.

With his family history and his natural curiosity, Dr. Fenker asked why we don't take a positive approach to living with Alzheimer's, one that is focused on helping people with the disease get the most out of life. And because Google has changed the way almost everyone uses memory today, what would Google for people with dementia be like? These questions became the springboard for his second book, *Don't Rain on My Parade: Living a Full Life with Alzheimer's and Dementia* (2017), and the invention of the MindPartner™ program.

MindPartner™ is a technology product that takes a rich set of memories and experiences from a person before the dementia is advanced, stores it online, and then gives it back over the full course of the dementia process in a collection of apps to support needs at different stages.

While writing *Don't Rain on My Parade* and interviewing people living with dementia, Dr. Fenker learned that the topic of death and choices around the end of life were highly important to this population, because every person knew that when the time came to make choices, they would not have any choices. Two friends living with dementia took their own lives during this period, fearing this eventual lack of control.

This, his newest book, *The Red Button*, grew out of these experiences plus the need, expressed by almost everyone in the dementia community, to gain access to hospice and possible options for an assisted death. This book furthers his interest in the disease and support for those with dementia and their caregivers.

Dr. Fenker is a National Science Foundation Fellow, was a member of the United States Gymnastics Team for six years (serving as Sport Psychologist and Science Director), was a consultant to the CIA, the Air Force, the Army, and the NSA, and represented the United States at two NATO conferences. He is a professional member of the International Alzheimer's Association and has served in several leadership roles with the Dementia Action Alliance.

He currently lives in Santa Fe, New Mexico, with his wife, Marilyn.

www.ingramcontent.com/pod-product-compliance
Ingram Content Group UK Ltd.
Pitfield, Milton Keynes, MK11 3LW, UK
UKHW020423250726
13967UKWH00007B/2792